The Complete Keto Air Fryer Cookbook #2019:

Easy, Lazy Keto Recipes & Recipes for Advanced Users

By Sam Bennett

I0415501

Contents

Introduction

The Ketogenic diet is a high-fat, moderate protein, and low-carb diet that transforms your body into a fat burning machine. The Ketogenic diet will show its benefits in only a few days, and it will help you lose weight, feel healthy and look amazing. You can follow the Ketogenic diet with an air fryer to prepare, quick, healthy, and delicious meals that trigger rapid weight loss and improve your overall health.

An air fryer offers a healthy cooking option for keto dieters and is the perfect tool to cook a wide range of keto-friendly foods, including breakfast, lunch, dinner, snacks, and even desserts. If you want delicious and easy to make Ketogenic air fryer recipes that your family can enjoy, then this cookbook is for you. These easy keto air fryer recipes are simple to make, taste delicious and provide a multitude of nutrients to keep you happy and healthy.

This Ketogenic air fryer cookbook is your go-to resource for making the Ketogenic diet a successful and enjoyable experience. Get a copy of this fantastic book and lose weight while taking much of the hard work out of cooking at the same time.

Recipe* - recipes for advanced users.

The Ketogenic Diet

The Ketogenic diet is a high fat, moderate protein, and low-carbohydrate diet regimen. There are two sources of fuel for the human body: carbohydrates/glucose/blood sugar and fat. When the body burns fat instead of glucose, molecules called ketone bodies are created, and these are what our body cells use for energy. The aim of the Ketogenic diet is to get the body to burn (metabolize) fat rather than glucose. Being a fat burner is referred to as being "in ketosis" or "keto-adapted," and it is the preferred metabolic state of the human body if you want to burn fat.

Most people believe that the carb-rich diet (glucose) is the only reliable source of fuel for the body. As a result, they became dependent on glucose. The truth is that fat is the ideal energy source and has been for most of human evolution. That is why we have all this fat on our bodies – to use when there is an emergency. We actually need only minimal amounts of glucose, most of which the liver can supply as needed on a daily basis.

The goal of the low-carb, high-fat Ketogenic diet is to get the body to use fat for fuel, not sugar. The Ketogenic diet is also moderate in protein.

The human body can't store protein, so it turns excess protein into glucose via a process called gluconeogenesis. This is why to keep glucose levels low; the Ketogenic diet calls for a moderate amount of protein. The theory behind the Ketogenic diet is that the body will rely on fat for energy instead of on carbohydrates, and, therefore, the body will become leaner as a result of having less fat stored in the body.

Ketosis

Ketosis is a metabolic process where your body burns deposits of fat instead of burning glucose. The word ketosis refers to the state of the human body when it lacks carbohydrates and starts to depend on fat for its energy. The aim of the Ketogenic diet is to reach the metabolic state of ketosis.

Air Fryer

An air fryer is a new cooking appliance that has become very popular. You can make all your favorite keto dishes in it. With an air fryer, you place the food inside, and the appliance circulates very hot air around the food and cooks it. Unlike a deep fryer, you need to use very little oil to air fry foods. So you get fried food with fewer calories. Besides frying, the air fryer can bake, grill, and roast foods.

The benefits of an air fryer

An air fryer offers more benefits to its users than one can really keep a count on. Here are the benefits of the air fryer:

1. Eat healthily: You can deep fry foods with an air fryer easily and eat healthily. You can use either a small amount of oil or no oil at all. You can cook a vast amount of foods in the air fryer including fries, chicken wings, onion rings and so on.
2. No waiting around: Waiting for your food to cook can be frustrating. An air fryer can fix this problem in absolutely no time. The fan inside the air fryer circulates very hot air, and the food is cooked very quickly.

3. You can cook anything you want: This is one of the best capabilities of the air fryer. The number of dishes you can cook in the air fryer is endless. You will enjoy grilled, stir-fried, broiled, roasted, fried, and baked food in the air fryer with just a press of a button. You can reheat frozen foods and leftovers.
4. The device is small: The device is tiny when compared to an oven, and you will save a lot of countertop space by using this device. The appliance is the same size as a coffee maker.
5. Easy to use and clean: The appliance is easy to use and easy to clean. Nobody loves to clean up the mess once they are done with the cooking. All you need to clean in an air fryer is a basket and a pan. Also, they are dishwasher friendly.
6. Saves money: The air fryer uses less energy to cook your favorite food. Unlike an oven, it doesn't heat up your entire house.

Buying guide for air fryers

1. Capacity: An air fryer comes in different sizes. The small air fryer ranges between 1 to 2 liters whereas the medium is 1.8 liters to 2.5 liters. The larger units of an air fryer are up to 5 liters and can be more. Choose one that meets your kitchen needs.

2. Wattage: A standard air fryer uses up to 1500 watts. However, watts vary from one model to another.
3. Temperature: The higher the temperature, the faster an air fryer will cook. This also means that it won't absorb much oil while cooking better, coated foods. Your air fryer should have easily navigable temperature control.
4. Safety: You need to choose an air fryer that is well-insulated and comes with proper safety measures to pull out the tray. Look for air fryers that won't slip off the kitchen countertop.

How to clean your air fryer?

1. Make sure your air fryer is unplugged and completely cool.
2. Use a damp cloth to wipe the outside.
3. Wash the basket, tray, and pan with hot water and dishwashing soap. Remember, all the removable parts of the air fryer are dishwasher safe.
4. Soak a sponge or a cloth with soapy hot water and clean the inside of the air fryer.
5. Clean any bits of food items with a brush.
6. Completely dry the basket, tray, and pan before putting them back into the air fryer.

Breakfast

Egg and Bacon Cups

Prep Time: 5 minutes	Cook Time: 15 minutes	Servings: 4

Ingredients

- Eggs – 4
- Bacon – 6 oz.
- Dried dill – ½ tsp.
- Paprika – 1 tsp.
- Salt – ½ tsp.

Directions

1. Preheat the air fryer to 360F.
2. Spray the inside of four ramekins with cooking oil.
3. Place the bacon in a way that it takes the shape of the bowl.
4. Crack an egg into each ramekin and place them inside the air fryer.
5. Cook for 15 minutes.
6. Once done, sprinkle with paprika, dried dill, and salt.
7. Serve.

Nutritional Facts Per Serving.

o   Calories: 350

o   Fat: 26g

o   Carb: 1g

o   Protein: 25g

Cheesy Spinach Omelette

Prep Time: 5 minutes	Cook Time: 8 minutes	Servings: 2

Ingredients

o   Large eggs – 4
o   Cheddar cheese – ½ cup, shredded
o   Fresh spinach – ½ cup chopped
o   Salt to taste

Directions

1. Whisk the eggs in a bowl. Place the eggs in the baking pan.
2. Stir in spinach and cheese and season with salt.

3. Preheat the air fryer to 380F and cook for 7 to 8 minutes.

Nutritional Facts Per Serving

o   Calories: 241

o   Fat: 18.1g

o   Carb: 1.3g

o   Protein: 18.3g

Sausage and Egg Breakfast Casserole

Prep Time: 5 minutes	Cook Time: 15 minutes	Servings: 3

Ingredients

o   Eggs – 6
o   Breakfast sausage – 1 lb. minced
o   Cheddar cheese – 2 cups, shredded
o   Sweet onion – 1, diced
o   Salt and pepper to taste
o   Oil to grease the dish

Directions

1. Grease a casserole dish with oil.
2. Place sausage onto the dish.
3. Whisk eggs and season with salt and pepper.
4. Pour the mixture into the casserole dish.
5. Spread the cheese on top.
6. Place the dish into the air fryer basket.
7. Cook at 360F for 15 minutes.
8. Serve.

Nutritional Facts Per Serving

o   Calories: 250

o   Fat: 13g

o   Carb: 1g

o   Protein: 18g

Eggs in Avocado Boats

Prep Time: 5 minutes	Cook Time: 6 minutes	Servings: 2

Ingredients

o   Avocado – 1 large, cut in halves and de-seeded
o   Eggs – 2
o   Salt and pepper to taste
o   Shredded cheddar – 1 cup

o   Parsley – 1 tsp.

Directions

1. Preheat the air fryer to 350F.
2. Crack the eggs in a bowl and mix them with the pulp of the avocado.
3. Add cheese, salt, and pepper.
4. Pour the mixture into the empty avocado.
5. Cook in the air fryer for 5 to 6 minutes.
6. Sprinkle with parsley and serve.

Nutritional Facts Per Serving

o   Calories: 450

o   Fat: 35g

o   Carb: 6g

o   Protein: 25g

Cheese Broccoli Quiche

Prep Time: 10 minutes	Cook Time: 10 minutes	Servings: 2

Ingredients

o   Eggs – 4
o   Cheddar cheese - 1 cup

- Broccoli – 1 cup, cooked
- Feta cheese – ¼ cup, crumbled
- Thyme – 1 tsp. dried
- Salt and pepper to taste

Directions

1. Whisk the eggs in a bowl with thyme, salt, and pepper.
2. Place broccoli in a quiche dish and add cheddar and feta.
3. Pour in the egg mixture.
4. Place the dish into the air fryer and cook 15 minutes at 360F.
5. Remove, slice and serve.

Nutritional Facts Per Serving

- Calories: 205

- Fat: 15g

- Carb: 0g

- Protein: 9g

Creamy Jalapeno Poppers

Prep Time: 5 minutes	Cook Time: 10 minutes	Servings: 2

Ingredients

- Salt – 1 tsp.
- Black pepper – ½ tsp.
- Sharp cheddar – ½ cup, shredded
- Cream cheese – 8 oz.
- Jalapeno peppers – 8, cut in half and deseeded

Directions

1. In a bowl, add cream cheese, black pepper, salt, and cheddar. Mix well.
2. Scoop the cream cheese mixture into the jalapenos.
3. Place the jalapenos into the air fryer basket and cook 10 minutes at 360F.
4. Serve.

Nutritional Facts Per Serving

- Calories: 50

- Fat: 5g

- Carb: 0g

o   Protein: 2.5g

Spinach and Egg Breakfast Frittata

Prep Time: 5 minutes	Cook Time: 10 to 12 minutes	Servings: 2

Ingredients

o   Small onion – 1, minced
o   Spinach – 1/3 pack (4 oz.)
o   Eggs – 3, beaten
o   Mozzarella cheese – 3 oz.
o   Olive oil – 1 Tbsp.
o   Salt and pepper to taste

Directions

1. Preheat the air fryer to 370F.
2. In a baking pan, heat the oil for 1 minute.
3. Add minced onion and cook for a couple of minutes.
4. Add spinach and cook until about half cooked, about 3 to 5 minutes.
5. In a large bowl, whisk the beaten eggs, season with salt and pepper and sprinkle with cheese. Pour mixture into a baking pan.

6. Place the pan in the air fryer and cook for 6 to 8 minutes or until cooked.

Nutritional Facts Per Serving

o   Calories: 361

o   Fat: 27.9g

o   Carb: 8.3g

o   Protein: 21.1g

Cheesy Egg Cups

Prep Time: 10 minutes	Cook Time: 10 minutes	Servings: 2

Ingredients

o   Eggs – 4
o   Chopped pickled jalapenos – ¼ cup
o   Full-fat cream cheese – 2 ounces
o   Shredded sharp cheddar cheese – ½ cup

Directions

1. Beat the eggs in a bowl, then pour into four silicon muffin cups.

2. In a bowl, place cream cheese, jalapenos, and cheddar. Microwave for 30 seconds and stir.
3. Take about ¼ of the mixture and place it in the center of one of the egg cups.
4. Repeat with the remaining mixture.
5. Place egg cups into the air fryer basket.
6. Set the time to 320F and Cook Time 10 minutes.
7. Serve.

Nutritional Facts Per Serving

o   Calories: 354

o   Fat: 25.3g

o   Carb: 2g

o   Protein: 21g

Breakfast Frittata*

Prep Time: 20 minutes	Cook Time:10 minutes	Servings: 2

Ingredients

o   Large eggs – 4
o   Unsweetened almond milk – ¼ cup

- o Italian sausage – ¼ pound
- o Cherry tomatoes – 4, cut in half
- o Chopped parsley – 2 Tbsp.
- o Salt and black pepper to taste
- o Olive oil – 1 Tbsp.

Directions

1. Place cut sausages and cherry tomatoes into the air fryer basket and cook at 360F for 3 to 5 minutes. Stir once.
2. Meanwhile, combine milk, eggs, and parsley in a bowl. Season with salt and pepper and whisk to mix.
3. Pour the egg mixture into the air fryer basket on top of the sausage and cook for 5 minutes more.
4. Enjoy.

Nutritional Facts Per Serving

- o Calories: 349

- o Fat: 27.9g

- o Carb: 7g

- o Protein: 16g

Hash Browns*

Prep Time: 20 minutes	Cook Time:12 minutes	Servings: 4

Ingredients

o Steamer cauliflower – 1 (12 ounce) bag
o Egg – 1
o Shredded sharp cheddar cheese – 1 cup

Directions

1. Cook the cauliflower in the microwave according to the package's instructions.
2. Cool and remove any excess moisture with a kitchen towel.
3. Mash cauliflower with a fork and add cheese and egg.
4. Cover the air fryer basket with parchment paper.
5. Take ¼ of the mixture and form it into a hash brown patty shape.
6. Place it onto the parchment and into the air fryer basket. Work in batches if necessary.
7. Set the temperature to 400F and cook for 12 minutes.
8. Flip the hash browns halfway through the cooking time.

9. Serve.

Nutritional Facts Per Serving

o   Calories: 153

o   Fat: 9.5g

o   Carb: 3.0g

o   Protein: 10.0g

Breakfast Muffins*

Prep Time: 10 minutes	Cook Time: 15 minutes	Servings: 6

Ingredients

o   Almond flour – 1 cup
o   Erythritol – ½ cup, powdered
o   Baking powder – ½ tsp.
o   Unsalted butter – ¼ cup, softened
o   Pure pumpkin puree – ¼ cup
o   Ground cinnamon – ½ tsp.
o   Ground nutmeg – ¼ tsp.
o   Vanilla extract – 1 tsp.
o   Egg – 2

Directions

1. Mix almond flour, butter, erythritol, baking powder, cinnamon, pumpkin puree, nutmeg, and vanilla in a bowl.
2. Gently stir in eggs.
3. Pour the batter into six muffin cups.
4. Place the muffin cups into the air fryer basket.
5. Adjust the temperature to 300F and set the timer for 15 minutes.
6. Cook and serve warm.

Nutritional Facts Per Serving

o Calories: 205

o Fat: 18g

o Carb: 3g

o Protein: 6.3g

Lunch

Fried Chicken

Prep Time: 5 minutes	Cook Time: 20 minutes	Servings: 8

Ingredients

o   Chicken wings – 8, whole
o   Chicken seasoning – 1 packet
o   Pepper – 1 Tbsp.
o   Olive oil – 1 Tbsp.

Directions

1. Marinate the chicken with chicken seasoning and pepper in a bowl.
2. Spray the chicken with olive oil and place in the air fryer basket.
3. Cook at 400F for 20 minutes. Flip the chicken at the 12 minute mark.
4. Serve.

Nutritional Facts Per Serving

o   Calories: 130

o   Fat: 7g

- o Carb: 1g

- o Protein: 10g

Parmesan Crusted Pork Chops

Prep Time: 6 minutes	Cook Time: 15 minutes	Servings: 4

Ingredients

- o Boneless pork chops – 1 ¼ lb.
- o Grated parmesan cheese – ½ cup
- o Egg – 1
- o Pork rinds – ½ cup, crushed
- o Lemon zest – ½ tsp.
- o Salt and pepper to taste

Directions

1. Pat dry the pork chops and season with salt and pepper.
2. Beat the eggs in a bowl.
3. Place parmesan cheese and crushed pork rinds on a large plate and pour the lemon zest onto it. Mix well.
4. Dip the pork chops into the egg, then coat with the parmesan mixture.

5. Place into the air fryer basket and cook at 380F for 15 minutes.
6. Flip the pork chops at the halfway mark.
7. Serve.

Nutritional Facts Per Serving

o Calories: 290

o Fat: 18g

o Carb: 1g

o Protein: 37g

Pecan Chicken Tender

Prep Time: 5 minutes	Cook Time: 12 minutes	Servings: 2

Ingredients

o Chicken tender - 1 lb.
o Finely crushed pecans – 1 cup
o Smoked paprika – ½ tsp.
o Sugar-free maple syrup – 2 Tbsp.
o Coarse ground mustard – ¼ cup
o Salt and pepper to taste

Directions

1. Season the chicken with salt, pepper, and paprika. Rub well.
2. Pour in mustard and syrup and mix well.
3. Place the crushed pecans onto a plate and roll the tenders to coat.
4. Place the tenders into the air fryer basket.
5. Cook at 350F for 12 minutes. Flip once.

Nutritional Facts Per Serving

o   Calories: 325

o   Fat: 3g

o   Carb: 6.5g

o   Protein: 28g

Zucchini Lasagna

Prep Time: 12 minutes	Cook Time: 25 minutes	Servings: 4

Ingredients

o   Marinara sauce – 1 cup
o   Zucchini – 1, thinly sliced

- o Italian sausage – ½ lb.
- o Shredded mozzarella cheese – 1 cup
- o Egg – 1

Directions

1. Spray a springform pan with oil.
2. Arrange the zucchini slices onto the bottom of the pan.
3. Pour ¼ cup of marinara sauce over the zucchini and spread evenly.
4. Add the sausage and spread evenly.
5. Top with the remaining sauce, followed by mozzarella cheese.
6. Cover the bowl with foil.
7. Cook at 350F for 20 minutes.
8. Then remove the foil and cook another 5 minutes.
9. Cool and serve.

Nutritional Facts Per Serving

- o Calories: 290

- o Fat: 8g

- o Carb: 4g

- o Protein: 15g

Cajun Salmon

Prep Time: 2 minutes	Cook Time: 12 minutes	Servings:1

Ingredients

- Salmon fillet – 1 (200g)
- Cajun seasoning – 1 Tbsp.
- Salt – ½ tsp.
- Lemon – 1

Directions

1. Preheat the air fryer to 350F.
2. Coat the salmon fillet with seasoning and salt. Rub well.
3. Place the salmon into the air fryer and cook for 12 minutes, keep the skin side on top.
4. Serve with a squeeze of lemon.

Nutritional Facts Per Serving

- Calories: 190

- Fat: 13g

- Carb: 0g

- Protein: 24g

Zesty Salmon Fillets

Prep Time: 5 minutes	Cook Time: 12 minutes	Servings: 4

Ingredients

- Crushed pork rind – ¾ cup
- Dry ranch-style dressing mix – 1 (30g) packet
- Olive oil – 2 ½ Tbsp.
- Eggs – 2, beaten
- Salmon fillets – 4
- Lemon wedges to garnish

Directions

1. Preheat the air fryer to 350F.
2. In a bowl, mix the ranch dressing and pork rinds. Add the oil and mix until mixed well.
3. Coat the fish fillets with the egg.
4. Then dip into the dry mixture and coat well.
5. Place into the air fryer carefully.
6. Cook for 12 to 13 minutes. Time depends on the thickness of the fillets.
7. Remove and serve.

Nutritional Facts Per Serving

- Calories 429

- Fat 23.1g

- Carb 5.3g

- Protein 40.4g

Chicken Parmesan

Prep Time: 5 minutes	Cook Time: 25 minutes	Servings: 4

Ingredients

- Chicken breast – 2 (about 8 oz. each) sliced to make 4 cutlets
- Pork rinds – 6 Tbsp.
- Grated Parmesan Cheese – 2 Tbsp.
- Butter – 1 Tbsp. melted
- Mozzarella cheese – 6 Tbsp.
- No-sugar add marinara – ½ cup
- Cooking spray

Directions

1. Preheat the air fryer 360F for 9 minutes. Grease the basket.

2. In a bowl, combine the Parmesan cheese and pork rinds.
3. Brush the chicken with the melted butter, then coat with the pork rind-cheese mixture.
4. Place the chicken in the air fryer and spray the top with oil.
5. Cook 6 minutes, then flip and top each with 1 ½ Tbsp. mozzarella and 1 Tbsp. sauce.
6. Cook until cheese is melted, about 3 more minutes.
7. Remove and repeat with the others.

Nutritional Facts Per Serving

o Calories 251

o Fat 9.5g

o Carb 4g

o Protein 31.5g

Ribeye Steak

Prep Time: 5 minutes	Cook Time: 14 minutes	Servings: 4

Ingredients

o Ribeye steak – 1 pound
o Steak rub – 1 Tbsp.
o Olive oil – 1 Tbsp.

Directions

1. Preheat the air fryer at 400F for 4 minutes.
2. Season the steak on both sides with olive oil and rub.
3. Place steak in the fry basket.
4. Cook at 400F for 14 minutes.
5. Flip the steak after 7 minutes.
6. When cooked, remove from the basket.
7. Let rest for 5 minutes. Slice and serve.

Nutritional Facts Per Serving

o Calories 344

o Fat 28.4g

o Carb 0.5g

o Protein 20g

Fried Shrimp with Sauce*

Prep Time: 10 minutes	Cook Time: 20 minutes	Servings: 4

Ingredients

- o Raw shrimp – 1 pound (peeled and deveined)
- o Egg white – 1
- o Almond flour – ½ cup
- o Pork rinds – ¾ cup, crushed
- o Paprika – 1 tsp.
- o Chicken seasoning to taste
- o Salt and pepper to taste
- o Cooking spray

Sauce

- o Greek yogurt – 1/3 cup
- o Keto Sriracha sauce – 2 Tbsp.
- o No sugar added chili sauce – ¼ cup

Directions

1. Preheat air fryer to 400F.
2. Season the shrimp with seasonings.
3. Place the pork rinds, egg whites, and flour in three separate bowls.

4. Dip the shrimp in the flour, then the egg whites and pork rinds.
5. Gently spray the shrimp with cooking spray, so they stay coated.
6. Add the shrimp to the air fryer basket.
7. Cook for 4 minutes, then flip and cook until crisp, about 4 minutes more.
8. To make the sauce, combine all the sauce ingredients and whisk to mix.

Nutritional Facts Per Serving

o   Calories 570

o   Fat 14.3g

o   Carb 4.9g

o   Protein 38g

Homemade Sausage Rolls*

Prep Time: 20 minutes	Cook Time: 25 minutes	Servings: 4

Ingredients

o   Almond flour – 225g
o   Butter – 100g

- o Olive oil – 1 Tbsp.
- o Sausage meat – 300g
- o Egg – 1, beaten
- o Mustard – 1 tsp.
- o Parsley – 1 tsp.
- o Salt and pepper

Directions

1. To make the pastry: in a bowl, place the butter, flour, and seasoning. Mix until the mixture resembles breadcrumbs. Bit by bit, add the olive oil and a little water and continue to mix the mixture until it becomes a flaky dough. Knead until it becomes smooth.
2. On a work surface, roll out the pastry and cut into a square shape. Rub the mustard into the pastry, place the sausage meat into the center, and brush the edges with egg. Roll up the sausage roll and divide into portions. Brush the top and sides of the rolls with more egg. Use a knife to slash the top of the sausage rolls.
3. Cook in the air fryer at 350F for 20 minutes. Then 5 minutes more at 400F. Flip once.
4. Serve.

Nutritional Facts Per Serving

- o Calories 488
- o Fat 46.9g
- o Carb 6.4g
- o Protein 22.2g

Crispy Pork Chops*

Prep Time: 5 minutes	Cook Time: 12 minutes	Servings: 6

Ingredients

- o Olive oil spray
- o Pork chops (without bones) – 6 (3/4 inch thick) 5 oz. each
- o Kosher salt
- o Egg – 1 large, beaten
- o Pork rinds – ½ cup
- o Almond flour – 1/3 cup
- o Parmesan cheese – 2 Tbsp. grated
- o Sweet paprika – 1 ¼ tsp.
- o Garlic powder – ½ tsp.
- o Onion powder – ½ tsp.
- o Chili powder – ¼ tsp.
- o Black pepper – 1/8 tsp.

Directions

1. Preheat the air fryer to 400F for 12 minutes and lightly grease the basket with oil.
2. Rub the pork chops with kosher salt.
3. In a bowl, combine black pepper, chili powder, onion powder, garlic powder, paprika, ¾ tsp. salt, parmesan cheese, almond flour, and pork rinds.
4. Place the beaten egg in another bowl. Coat the pork into the egg and then in the dry mixture.
5. Place 3 chops in the basket and spray with oil.
6. Cook for 12 minutes. Flip at the 6 minute mark and spray both sides with oil.
7. Repeat with the remaining pork and serve.

Nutritional Facts Per Serving

o Calories 378

o Fat 13g

o Carb 4g

o Protein 33g

Dinner

Sriracha Chicken Wings

Prep Time: 3 minutes	Cook Time: 20 minutes	Servings: 2

Ingredients

o   Chicken wings – 1 lb.
o   Sriracha sauce – 2 Tbsp.
o   Liquid aminos – 1 ½ Tbsp.

Directions

1. Preheat the air fryer to 360F.
2. Spray the air fryer basket with cooking oil.
3. Add sriracha and liquid aminos in a bowl.
4. Toss the chicken wings into the sauce mixture and coat evenly.
5. Place the coated chicken into the air fryer and cook for 20 minutes.
6. Flip the chicken at the 12 minute mark.
7. Serve.

Nutritional Facts Per Serving

o   Calories 265

o   Fat 13g

- Carb 0.8g

- Protein 34g

Beef-Stuffed Zucchini

Prep Time: 5 minutes	Cook Time: 13 minutes	Servings: 4

Ingredients

- Zucchini – 2 large, cut in half lengthwise
- Ground beef – 1 lb.
- Shredded cheddar – ½ cup

Directions

1. Scoop the pulp out of the zucchini, leaving about 1/4.
2. Place the ground beef into the zucchini, covering the gap.
3. Place into the air fryer basket and cook at 400F for 10 minutes.
4. Then add the shredded cheddar onto the zucchini and cook for another 4 minutes.
5. Serve and enjoy.

Nutritional Facts Per Serving

- o Calories 150

- o Fat 10g

- o Carb 1g

- o Protein 10g

Marinated Steak

Prep Time: 12 minutes	Cook Time: 6 minutes	Servings: 4

Ingredients

- o New York Strip Steaks – 2
- o Liquid aminos – 1 Tbsp.
- o Steak seasoning – 1 Tbsp.
- o Cocoa powder – ½ Tbsp.
- o Liquid smoke – 1 tsp.
- o Salt and pepper to taste

Directions

1. Drizzle the liquid aminos and liquid smoke onto the steaks.
2. Add the seasonings and rub well. Marinate in the refrigerator for 10 minutes.

3. Place the steaks into the air fryer and cook at 350F for 6 minutes. Cooking time varies depending on the thickness.
4. Serve.

Nutritional Facts Per Serving

o Calories 234

o Fat 14g

o Carb 0.5g

o Protein 25g

Spicy Lamb Steak

Prep Time: 15 minutes	Cook Time: 15 minutes	Servings: 4

Ingredients

o Boneless lamb sirloin steak – 1 lb.
o Cayenne – 1 tsp.
o Garam masala – 1 tsp.
o Garlic – 5 cloves
o Ground fennel – 1 tsp.

Directions

1. Except for the lamb, add all the ingredients in a blender and blend finely.
2. Place the lamb into a bowl and rub with the blended mixture. Mix and marinate for 10 minutes.
3. Cook the lamb steaks at 330F for 15 minutes.
4. Flip once at the 10 minute mark.

Nutritional Facts Per Serving

o   Calories 150

o   Fat 2g

o   Carb 2g

o   Protein 24g

Lemon Pepper Chicken

Prep Time: 4 minutes	Cook Time: 18 minutes	Servings: 1

Ingredients

o   Chicken breast – 4 oz.
o   Chicken seasoning – 1 Tbsp.
o   Lemon – 2, juiced
o   Black peppercorns – 2 Tbsp.

- Salt and pepper to taste
- Garlic puree – 1 tsp.

Directions

1. Preheat the air fryer to 350F.
2. In aluminum foil, add all the ingredients, except salt and pepper.
3. Rub the chicken breast with salt and pepper on both sides.
4. Place the chicken breast in the aluminum foil and coat it well with the ingredients.
5. Close the aluminum foil tightly and use a rolling pin's blunt end to flatten the chicken breast.
6. Cook for 18 minutes.
7. Serve hot.

Nutritional Facts Per Serving

- Calories 120

- Fat 4g

- Carb 2.5g

- Protein 24g

Bacon Wrapped Chicken

Prep Time: 5 minutes	Cook Time: 15 minutes	Servings: 2

Ingredients

o   Chicken tender – 1 pound, skinless and boneless
o   Bacon strips – 4 to 6
o   Erythritol – 4 Tbsp. powdered
o   Chili powder – ½ tsp.

Directions

1. In a bowl, mix the erythritol and chili powder.
2. Cut chicken tenders into 2-inch pieces.
3. Wrap chicken pieces with the bacon strips and mix in the chili mixture.
4. Preheat the air fryer to 390 to 400F.
5. Place wrapped chicken into the air fryer and cook for 10 to 15 minutes. The time depends on the size of the chicken.
6. Serve.

Nutritional Facts Per Serving

o   Calories 538

o   Fat 28.9g

- Carb 8g

- Protein 63.6g

Chicken Patties

Prep Time: 5 minutes	Cook Time: 15 minutes	Servings: 4

Ingredients

- Chicken breasts - 1 pound
- Pumpkin – 1 cup, pureed
- Carrot – 1 small, sliced
- Medium onion – 1, sliced
- Almond or coconut flour – 1 cup
- Vinegar – 3 Tbsp.
- Garlic powder – 1 tsp.
- Chili powder – ½ tsp.
- Salt and black pepper to taste

Directions

1. Cut chicken into long slices. Season with garlic powder, salt, and pepper. Drizzle with vinegar and set aside for 30 minutes.

2. Mix the rest of the ingredients in a bowl and add the marinated chicken. Stir to combine.
3. Roll chicken patties with your hands and cook at 360F in the air fryer for 8 to 15 minutes, or until brown and crispy. Flip once.

Nutritional Facts Per Serving

o   Calories 308

o   Fat 22.3g

o   Carb 4.7g

o   Protein 25g

Fried Turkey Breast

Prep Time: 10 minutes	Cook Time: 25 minutes	Servings: 6

Ingredients

o   Turkey breast – 5 pounds, skinless and boneless
o   Salt – 2 tsp.
o   Black pepper – 1 tsp.
o   Dried cumin – ½ tsp.
o   Olive oil – 2 Tbsp.

Directions

1. Rub the whole turkey breast with seasoning and olive oil.
2. Preheat the air fryer to 340F and cook a turkey breast for 15 minutes. Then flip and cook until crispy, about 10 to 15 minutes more.
3. Slice and serve with vegetables.

Nutritional Facts Per Serving

o Calories 330

o Fat 6.4g

o Carb 1g

o Protein 64g

Coconut Shrimp*

Prep time: 10 minutes	Cook time: 14 minutes	Servings: 4

Ingredients

- Large shrimp – 1 pound, about 16 to 20, peeled and deveined
- Almond flour – ½ cup
- Egg whites – 2
- Pork rinds – ½ cup, crushed
- Shredded unsweetened coconut – ½ cup
- Zest of one lime
- Salt – ½ tsp.
- Cayenne pepper – ¼ tsp.
- Ground black pepper as needed
- Duck sauce for serving

Directions

1. Place the flour in a bowl, and season well with salt and black pepper.
2. Whisk the eggs in another bowl.
3. Combine the cayenne pepper, salt, lime zest, coconut and pork rinds in another bowl.
4. Preheat the air fryer to 400F.
5. Dredge each shrimp first in the flour, then dip it in the egg mixture, and finally press it into the coconut-pork rind mixture to coat all sides.
6. Place the coated shrimp on a plate and spray on all sides with oil.
7. Air-fry the shrimp in two batches. Do not overcrowd the basket.

8. Air fry at 400F for 5 to 6 minutes, or until the shrimp is firm when you squeeze it gently. Shake once. Repeat with the second batch of shrimp.

9. Lower the temperature to 340F. Place the first batch of shrimp into the basket with the second batch already in the basket and air fry for 2 more minutes.

10. Serve with duck sauce.

Nutritional Facts Per Serving

o Calories 179

o Fat 8.4g

o Carb 2.4g

o Protein 23.9g

Fried Fishcakes*

Prep Time: 10 minutes	Cook Time: 15 minutes	Servings: 4

Ingredients

o Any white fish – 1 pound, boneless and cooked

- Cauliflower florets – 1 cup, cooked and mashed
- Coconut milk – 3 Tbsp.
- Unsalted butter – 3 Tbsp.
- Almond flour – 2 Tbsp.
- Freshly chopped dill – 1 Tbsp.
- Freshly chopped parsley – 1 Tbsp.
- Salt – 1 pinch
- Black pepper – ¼ tsp. ground

Directions

1. Combine cooked fish, mashed cauliflower and chopped herbs. Season with salt and pepper and mix.
2. Add the butter and milk until you have a nice consistency. Add a little flour and then make patty cakes with your hands.
3. Keep in the refrigerator for 1 hour to make them solid.
4. In the air fryer, cook fishcakes at 390F for 12 to 15 minutes, or until golden. Flip once.
5. Serve with veggies.

Nutritional Facts Per Serving

- Calories 405

- Fat 39g

- Carb 2.1g

- Protein 13.4g

Baby Back Ribs*

Prep Time: 5 minutes	Cook Time: 30 minutes	Servings: 4

Ingredients

- Toasted sesame oil – 1 Tbsp.
- Liquid aminos – 1 Tbsp.
- Dry white wine – 1 Tbsp.
- Liquid stevia – 1 Tbsp.
- Minced garlic – 1 tsp.
- Minced fresh ginger – 1 tsp.
- Baby back ribs – 1 (1 ½ pound), cut into individual ribs

Directions

1. Except for the ribs, combine all the ingredients in a bowl. Add the ribs and coat well. Cover and marinate at room temperature for 30 minutes.
2. Discard the marinade and cook in the air fryer for 350F for 30 minutes. Shake twice.

Nutritional Facts Per Serving

o   Calories 434

o   Fat 37.2g

o   Carb 0.3g

o   Protein 22.5g

Snacks and Side Dishes

Chicken Kebab

Prep Time: 15 minutes	Cook Time: 15 minutes	Servings: 6

Ingredients

o Boneless chicken breast - 1.5 lb. cut into bite-sized pieces
o Smoked paprika – ½ tsp.
o Turmeric – 1 tsp.
o Ground black pepper – ½ tsp.
o Plain Greek yogurt – ¼ cup

Directions

1. In a blender, place turmeric, black pepper, smoked paprika, and Greek yogurt. Blend until smooth.
2. Pour mixture over the chicken and coat evenly.
3. Marinate the chicken for 15 minutes.
4. Place the chicken into the air fryer basket.
5. Cook at 370F for 15 minutes. Flip the chicken after 8 minutes.
6. Serve.

Nutritional Facts Per Serving

o   Calories 150

o   Fat 2g

o   Carb 0.5g

o   Protein 20g

Zucchini Parmesan Chips

Prep Time: 4 minutes	Cook Time: 10 minutes	Servings: 4

Ingredients

o   Zucchini – 2, thinly sliced
o   Egg – 1
o   Pork rinds – ½ cup crushed
o   Parmesan – ½ cup, grated
o   Smoked paprika – ½ tsp.
o   Salt and pepper to taste

Directions

1. Beat eggs with salt and pepper in a bowl. In another bowl, mix grated cheese, smoked paprika, and pork rinds.

2. Dip the zucchini slice into the egg mixture, then the pork rinds mixture. Coat well.
3. Spray the coated zucchini slices with cooking spray.
4. Place into the air fryer basket; do not overlap.
5. Cook at 350F for 8 minutes. Flip once.
6. Serve.

Nutritional Facts Per Serving

o Calories 40

o Fat 3g

o Carb 1g

o Protein 1g

Cheese Stuffed Mushroom

Prep Time: 6 minutes	Cook Time: 8 minutes	Servings: 5

Ingredients

o Large mushrooms – 8 oz. stem cut
o Parmesan – ¼ cup, shredded
o Cream cheese – 4 oz.

- o Worcestershire sauce – 1 tsp.
- o Cheddar cheese – 1/8 cup
- o Salt and pepper to taste

Directions

1. Combine the cheddar, parmesan, cream cheese, sauce, salt, and pepper in a bowl. Mix well.
2. Stuff the mixture into the mushrooms.
3. Place the mushrooms into the air fryer and cook for 8 minutes at 370F.
4. Serve.

Nutritional Facts Per Serving

- o Calories 105
- o Fat 9g
- o Carb 2g
- o Protein 9g

Bacon Wrapped Chicken

Prep Time: 10 minutes	Cook Time: 13 minutes	Servings: 4

Ingredients

- Chicken breast – 1 lb. cut into cubes
- Bacon – 6 slices, cut into thirds
- Chili powder – ½ Tbsp.
- Cayenne pepper – 1/8 tsp.
- Salt to taste

Directions

1. Place a piece of chicken onto a piece of bacon. Roll it up and secure with a toothpick.
2. Mix the salt, chili powder, and cayenne pepper into a bowl.
3. Coat the bacon wrapped chicken into the mixture.
4. Place the bacon wrapped chicken into the air fryer basket and cook at 380F for 13 minutes.
5. Serve.

Nutritional Facts Per Serving

- Calories 120

- Fat 10g

- Carb 0g

- Protein 18g

Buffalo Cauliflower

Prep Time: 5 minutes	Cook Time: 10 minutes	Servings: 4

Ingredients

o   Cauliflower florets – 4 cups
o   Pork rinds – 1 cup, crushed
o   Sea salt – 1 tsp.
o   Butter – ¼ cup, melted
o   No sugar added buffalo sauce – ¼ cup

Directions

1. Melt the butter in a bowl.
2. Add the sauce and stir to mix. Mix the pork rinds and salt in another bowl.
3. Dip each floret into the buffalo mixture and coat well.
4. Then dip into the pork rind mixture.
5. Place the floret into the air fryer and cook at 350F for 10 minutes.
6. Shake the florets after 5 minutes.
7. Serve.

Nutritional Facts Per Serving

o   Calories 160

o   Fat 4g

- Carb 3g

- Protein 1g

Perfect Brussels Sprouts

Prep Time: 5 minutes	Cook Time: 10 minutes	Servings: 2

Ingredients

- Brussels sprouts – 2 cups (sliced in half lengthwise)
- Olive oil – 1 Tbsp.
- Balsamic vinegar – 1 Tbsp.
- Sea salt – ¼ tsp.

Directions

1. Toss together the Brussels Sprouts, vinegar, salt, and oil in a bowl.
2. Air fry at 400F for 8 to 10 minutes. Shake the bowl after 5 minutes and at the 8-minute mark.
3. Enjoy!

Nutritional Facts Per Serving

- o Calories 100

- o Fat 7.3g

- o Carb 6.1g

- o Protein 3g

Butter Roasted Radishes

Prep Time: 10 minutes	Cook Time: 10 minutes	Servings: 4

Ingredients

- o Radishes – 1 pound, cut into quarters
- o Unsalted butter – 2 Tbsp. melted
- o Garlic powder – ½ tsp.
- o Dried parsley – ½ tsp.
- o Dried oregano – ¼ tsp.
- o Ground black pepper – ¼ tsp.

Directions

1. Add butter and seasoning in a bowl. Toss radishes in the bowl to coat well.

2. Place the coated radishes into the air fryer basket.
3. Set the temperature to 350F and cook for 10 minutes.
4. Toss the radishes at the 5-minute mark.
5. Serve warm.

Nutritional Facts Per Serving

- Calories 63

- Fat 5.4g

- Carb 1.6g

- Protein 1g

Buffalo Cauliflower

Prep Time: 5 minutes	Cook Time: 5 minutes	Servings: 4

Ingredients

- Cauliflower florets – 4 cups
- Salted butter – 2 Tbsp. melted
- Dry ranch seasoning – ½ (1-ounce) packet
- Buffalo sauce – ¼ cup

Directions

1. Toss the cauliflower with the butter and dry ranch in a bowl. Place into the air fryer basket.
2. Set the temperature to 400F and cook for 5 minutes.
3. Shake the basket two to three times during cooking.
4. Remove from the air fryer and toss in buffalo sauce.
5. Serve warm.

Nutritional Facts Per Serving

o Calories 87

o Fat 5.6g

o Carb 3.2g

o Protein 2.1g

Chicken Tenders*

Prep Time: 10 minutes	Cook Time: 13 minutes	Servings: 4

Ingredients

- Eggs – 2 large
- Garlic powder – 2 tsp.
- Salt – 1 tsp.
- Ground black pepper – ½ tsp.
- Pork rinds – ¾ cup, crushed
- Shredded unsweetened coconut – ¾ cup
- Chicken tenders – 1 pound (about 8 tenders)
- Cooking spray

Directions

1. Preheat your air fryer to 450F.
2. In a bowl, add the eggs and season with salt, pepper and garlic powder. Mix well. In another bowl, add coconut and pork rinds. Stir to mix.
3. Dip the chicken in egg mixture and coat well, then dip into the dry mixture. Coat well.
4. Place the coated chicken in the greased basket. Spray with cooking spray.
5. Bake until the coating is crisp and golden brown, and chicken is cooked, about 12 to 14 minutes. Shake once.

Nutritional Facts Per Serving

- Calories 242

- Fat 6.7

- Carb 6.7

- Protein 28.8

Pork Rind Tortillas*

Prep Time: 10 minutes	Cook Time: 5 minutes	Servings: 4

Ingredients

- Pork rinds – 1 ounce
- Shredded mozzarella cheese – ¾ cup
- Full-fat cream cheese – 2 Tbsp.
- Egg – 1

Directions

1. Pulse pork rinds in a food processor until finely ground.
2. Place mozzarella into a bowl. Break cream cheese into small pieces and add them to the bowl.
3. Microwave for 30 seconds, or until both types of cheese are melted and can easily be stirred together into a ball.

4. Add ground pork rinds and egg to the cheese mixture.
5. Continue stirring until the mixture forms a ball. If it cools too much, microwave for 10 more seconds.
6. Separate the dough into four small balls.
7. Place each ball of dough between two sheets of parchment and roll into a ¼ flat layer.
8. Place tortillas into the air fryer basket in a single layer.
9. Set the temperature to 400F and cook for 5 minutes.
10. Serve.

Nutritional Facts Per Serving

o Calories 145

o Fat 10g

o Carb 1g

o Protein 10.7g

Prosciutto-Wrapped Asparagus*

Prep Time: 10 minutes	Cook Time: 10 minutes	Servings: 4

Ingredients

o   Asparagus – 1 pound
o   Prosciutto – 12 (0.5 ounce) slices
o   Coconut oil – 1 Tbsp. melted
o   Lemon juice – 2 tsp.
o   Red pepper flakes – 1/8 tsp.
o   Grated Parmesan cheese – 1/3 cup
o   Salted butter – 2 Tbsp. melted

Directions

1. On a clean work surface, place an asparagus spear onto a slice of prosciutto.
2. Drizzle with lemon juice and coconut oil.
3. Sprinkle Parmesan and red pepper flakes across asparagus.
4. Roll prosciutto around an asparagus spear.
5. Place into the air fryer basket.
6. Set temperature to 375F and cook for 10 minutes.

7. Drizzle the asparagus roll with butter before serving.

Nutritional Facts Per Serving

o   Calories 263

o   Fat 20.2g

o   Carb 4.3g

o   Protein 13.9g

Dessert

Cheesecake Bites

Prep Time: 5 minutes	Cook Time: 7 minutes	Servings: 2

Ingredients

- o   Cream cheese – 8 oz. softened
- o   Erythritol – ½ cup, plus 2 Tbsp.
- o   Vanilla extract – ½ tsp.
- o   Almond flour – ½ cup
- o   Heavy cream – ½ packet

Directions

1. Mix the cream cheese with ½ packet heavy cream, ½-cup erythritol, and vanilla extract until smooth.
2. Scoop the mixture onto a parchment paper-lined baking sheet.
3. Freeze 30 minutes for best results.
4. Mix the almond flour with 2 Tbsp. erythritol in a bowl.
5. Roll the frozen bites into the almond flour mixture.

6. Place the cheesecake bites into the air fryer basket and cook for 7 minutes at 370F.

Nutritional Facts Per Serving

o   Calories 110

o   Fat 7g

o   Carb 1g

o   Protein 2g

Brownies

Prep Time: 10 minutes	Cook Time: 20 minutes	Servings: 6

Ingredients

o   Almond flour – ½ cup
o   Powdered erythritol – ½ cup
o   Unsweetened cocoa powder – 2 Tbsp.
o   Baking powder – ½ tsp.
o   Unsalted butter – ¼ cup, softened
o   Egg – 1
o   Chopped pecans – ¼ cup
o   Sugar-free chocolate chips – ¼ cup

Directions

1. Mix almond flour, baking powder, cocoa powder, and erythritol in a bowl.
2. Stir in egg and butter.
3. Fold in chocolate chips and pecans.
4. Scoop mixture into a baking pan and place the pan into the air fryer basket.
5. Cook at 300F for 20 minutes.
6. Cool, sliced and serve.

Nutritional Facts Per Serving

o Calories 215

o Fat 18.9g

o Carb 2.3g

o Protein 4.2g

Mug Cake

Prep Time: 5 minutes	Cook Time: 25 minutes	Servings: 1

Ingredients

o Egg – 1

- Coconut flour – 2 Tbsp.
- Heavy whipping cream – 2 Tbsp.
- Granular erythritol – 2 Tbsp.
- Vanilla extract – ¼ tsp.
- Baking powder – ¼ tsp.

Directions

1. Whisk egg in a 4-inch ramekin. Then add the remaining ingredients and mix. Stir until smooth.
2. Place into the air fryer basket.
3. Cook at 300F for 25 minutes.
4. Serve.

Nutritional Facts Per Serving

- Calories 237

- Fat 16.4g

- Carb 5.7g

- Protein 9.9g

Chocolate Chip Cookie

Prep time: 7 minutes	Cook time: 9 minutes	Servings: 4

Ingredients

o   Softened butter – 3 Tbsp.
o   Erythritol – ¼ cup plus 1 Tbsp. powdered
o   Egg yolk – 1
o   Almond flour – ½ cup
o   Ground white chocolate – 2 Tbsp. no sugar added
o   Baking soda – ¼ tsp.
o   Vanilla – ½ tsp.
o   Chocolate chips – ¾ cup, no sugar added

Directions

1. In a medium bowl, beat the butter and erythritol together until fluffy. Stir in egg yolk.
2. Add the vanilla, baking soda, white chocolate, and flour. Mix well. Stir in the chocolate chips.
3. Line a (6-by-6-by-2 inch) baking pan with the parchment paper. Spray the parchment paper with nonstick baking spray.
4. Spread the batter into the prepared pan, leaving a ½-inch border on all sides.
5. Bake at 300F for 9 minutes or until the cookie is lightly brown and just barely set.

6. Remove the pan from the air fryer and let cook for 10 minutes.
7. Remove the cookie from the pan, remove the parchment paper and let cool on a wire rack.

Nutritional Facts Per Serving

o Calories 362

o Fat 27.3g

o Carb 4g

o Protein 6g

Chocolate Cake

Prep time: 10 minutes	Cook time: 25 minutes	Servings: 6

Ingredients

o Eggs – 3
o Sour cream – ½ cup
o Almond flour – 1 cup
o Erythritol – 2/3 cup, powdered
o Butter – 1 stick, room temperature
o Cocoa powder – 1/3 cup

- o Baking powder – 1 tsp.
- o Baking soda – ½ tsp.
- o Vanilla – 2 tsp.

Directions

1. Preheat air fryer to 320F.
2. Mix the wet ingredients in a bowl and dry ingredients in another.
3. Gradually pour the dry mixture into the wet. Lightly mix.
4. Place in the air fryer basket.
5. Cook for 25 minutes.
6. Check if the cake is done; if not, then cook for another 5 minutes.
7. Cool on a wire rack.

Nutritional Facts Per Serving

- o Calories 321
- o Fat 30.8g
- o Carb 7.2g
- o Protein 7.7g

Lemon Tarts

Prep time: 10 minutes	Cook time: 15 minutes	Servings: 4

Ingredients

o   Butter – ½ cup
o   Almond flour – ½ pound
o   Erythritol – 3 Tbsp. powdered
o   Lemon – 1 large (juice and zest)
o   Lemon curd – 2 Tbsp.
o   Nutmeg – 1 pinch

Directions

1. In a bowl, combine erythritol, almond flour, and butter. Mix until it looks like breadcrumbs. Then add lemon zest and juice, and cinnamon and mix again. If needed, add 2 Tbsp. water to make a soft dough.
2. Sprinkle pastry tins with almond flour. Add dough and top with lemon zest.
3. Preheat the air fryer to 360F and cook mini lemon tarts for 15 minutes or until ready.
4. Serve.

Nutritional Facts Per Serving

o   Calories 304

- Fat 29.9g

- Carb 8.6g

- Protein 2.9g

Coconut Cookies

Prep time: 5 minutes	Cook time: 12 minutes	Servings: 10

Ingredients

- Egg – 1
- Dried coconut – 3 Tbsp.
- Butter – 3 oz.
- Erythritol – 2 oz. powdered
- Vanilla extract – 1 tsp.
- Chocolate – 2 oz. no sugar added
- Almond flour – 5 oz.

Directions

1. In a bowl, beat butter and erythritol until fluffy.
2. Add one egg, vanilla extract and stir to combine.

3. Crush the chocolate into small pieces. Add them to the mixture.
4. Roll small balls with hands.
5. Roll these balls in the dried coconut.
6. Place balls onto the baking sheet.
7. Preheat the air fryer to 370F.
8. Bake coconut balls for 8 minutes. Shake once.
9. Lower temperature to 280 to 300F and cook for 4 minutes more.
10. Serve.

Nutritional Facts Per Serving

o   Calories 206

o   Fat 18.6g

o   Carb 6.7g

o   Protein 4.8g

Fried Cheesecake Bites

Prep Time: 5 minutes	Cook Time: 2 minutes	Servings: 16

Ingredients

- Cream cheese – 8 ounces, softened
- Erythritol – ½ cup, powdered
- Cream – 2 Tbsp. divided
- Vanilla extract – ½ tsp.
- Almond flour – ½ cup
- Erythritol – 2 Tbsp.

Directions

1. Mix heavy cream, vanilla, erythritol, and cream cheese until smooth.
2. Line a baking sheet with parchment paper and drop scoops of mixture on it.
3. Freeze until firm, about 30 minutes.
4. Mix 2 Tbsp. erythritol with almond flour in a bowl.
5. Dip the bites into the 2 Tbsp. cream, then coat into the flour mixture.
6. Cook in the air fryer at 350F for 2 minutes.
7. Serve.

Nutritional Facts Per Serving

- Calories 80

- Fat 7g

- Carb 2g

- Protein 2g

Marble Cake*

Prep time: 5 minutes	Cook time: 17 minutes	Servings: 6

Ingredients

- Erythritol - 7 Tbsp. powdered
- Almond flour – ½ cup
- Eggs – 4, whisked
- Baking powder – 1 tsp.
- Cocoa powder – 5 tsp.
- Butter – 2/3 cup, melted
- Lime juice – ½ tsp.

Directions

1. Preheat the air fryer to 356F.
2. Mix 3 Tbsp. of melted butter with the cocoa powder to form a paste.
3. Add the erythritol to the remaining butter and mix well. Stir in the eggs, almond flour, and baking powder and mix until smooth. Pour in the lime and stir.
4. Place a greased baking pan into the air fryer and allow to heat for a minute.

5. Pour some of the batter into the hot pan, then add a layer of the chocolate mixture, then the batter, chocolate and lastly, top with batter. Use a skewer to create a swirl.
6. Place in the air fryer and bake for 17 minutes.

Nutritional Facts Per Serving

o Calories 277

o Fat 27.9g

o Carb 3.5g

o Protein 5.9g

Cheesecake Brownies*

Prep Time: 20 minutes	Cook Time: 35 minutes	Servings: 6

Ingredients

o Almond flour – ½ cup
o Powdered erythritol – 1 cup, divided
o Unsweetened cocoa powder – 2 Tbsp.
o Baking powder – ½ tsp.
o Unsalted butter – ¼ cup, softened

- Eggs – 2, divided
- Full-fat cream cheese – 8 ounces, softened
- Heavy whipping cream – ¼ cup
- Vanilla extract – 1 tsp.
- No-sugar-added peanut butter – 2 Tbsp.

Directions

1. In a bowl, mix ½ cup erythritol, almond flour, baking powder, and cocoa powder. Stir in one egg and butter.
2. Scoop mixture into a 6-inch round baking pan.
3. Place pan into the air fryer basket.
4. Cook at 300F for 20 minutes.
5. In a bowl, beat the remaining ½-cup erythritol, cream cheese, heavy cream, peanut butter, vanilla, and remaining egg until fluffy.
6. Pour mixture over cooled brownies.
7. Place pan back into the air fryer basket.
8. Cook at 300F for 15 minutes.
9. Cool, then refrigerate for 2 hours before serving.

Nutritional Facts Per Serving

- Calories 347

- Fat 30.9g

- o Carb 3.8g

- o Protein 8.3g

Mini Cheesecake*

Prep Time: 10 minutes	Cook Time: 15 minutes	Servings: 2

Ingredients

- o Walnuts – ½ cup
- o Salted butter – 2 Tbsp.
- o Granular erythritol – 2 Tbsp.
- o Full-fat cream cheese – 4 ounces, softened
- o Egg – 1
- o Vanilla extract – ½ tsp.
- o Powdered erythritol – 1/8 cup

Directions

1. Place granular erythritol, butter, and walnuts in a food processor. Pulse until a dough forms.
2. Press dough into a 4-inch springform pan and place the pan into the air fryer basket.
3. Cook at 400F for 5 minutes.

4. Remove and cool.
5. In a bowl, mix egg, cream cheese, powdered erythritol, and vanilla extract until smooth.
6. Spoon mixture on top of baked walnut crust and place into the air fryer basket.
7. Cook at 300F for 10 minutes.
8. Chill for 2 hours and serve.

Nutritional Facts Per Serving

o   Calories 531

o   Fat 48.3g

o   Carb 5.1g

o   Protein 11.4g

About the Author

Sam Bennett is a writer, wellness expert in nutrition and professional cook. He is the author of several cookbooks. Sam is a passionate advocate for the Ketogenic diet lifestyle. He understands the connection between food and how it makes us all feel inside and out. His mission is to prove to the world that special diets need not be boring or restrictive and that low-carb and gluten-free dishes can be just as good or better than their conventional counterparts. After struggling with his weight throughout his childhood, he decided to study health and wellness. Sam discovered the Keto diet and decided to give it a shot with amazing weight loss results. Sam's focus is on easy-to-make low-carb and gluten-free comfort food. Sam has devoted his career to helping others to stay fit and feel good on the Ketogenic diet. Sam's passion is reaching out to others who struggle with body weight and helping them to learn why a Ketogenic diet works. He loves to challenge himself on a daily basis and draws inspiration from family and friends. His strong passion for healthy living, dieting, nutrition, and weight loss has led to his successful transformation. He is passionate about cooking; sharing his experience to help others, and enjoying life to the last drop. Sam lives in the San Francisco Bay Area with his two children and loving wife Megan.

Conclusion

Nowadays a Ketogenic diet is the most effective and easy to follow diet around the world. Not only will it help you lose weight fast, but it will also make you feel better, improve mood, boost energy, and make you healthy. If you are ready to turn your life around for the better, then this cookbook will help you understand the fundamentals of the Ketogenic diet and provide you easy and delicious air fryer recipes that your whole family will enjoy.

Please, leave an honest review

https://www.amazon.com/Complete-Keto-Fryer-Cookbook-2019-ebook/dp/B07QPWJ61J

www.ingramcontent.com/pod-product-compliance
Lightning Source LLC
Chambersburg PA
CBHW032103280526
45784CB00013B/3005